P9-DTW-441

GREAT BRAIDS!

THE NEW WAY TO EXCITING HAIRSTYLES

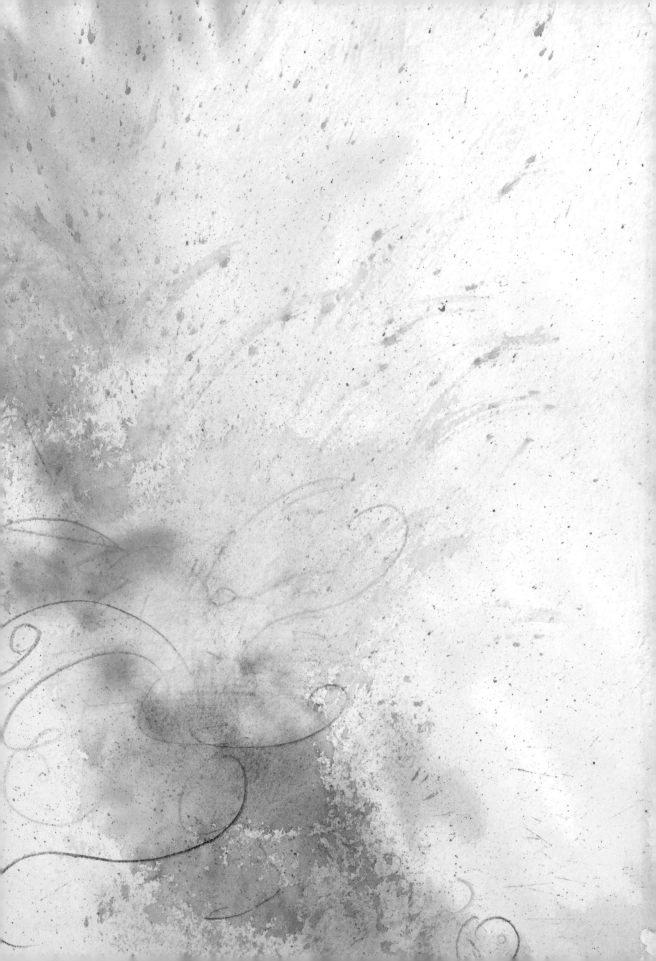

GREAT BRAIDS!

THE NEW WAY TO EXCITING HAIRSTYLES

THOMAS HARDY

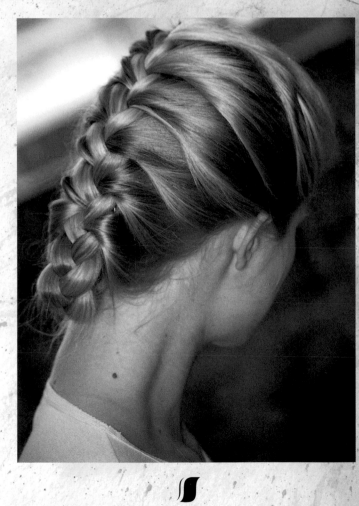

FEB 2 0 1998

Sterling Publishing Co., Inc. New York
A Sterling/Chapelle Book

FOR CHAPELLE LTD.

Owner: Jo Packham

Editor: Karmen Quinney

Staff: Marie Barber, Malissa Boatwright, Kass Burchett, Rebecca Christensen, Holly Fuller, Marilyn Goff, Michael Hannah, Shirley Heslop, Holly Hollingsworth, Susan Jorgensen, Susan Laws, Barbara Milburn, Leslie Ridenour, Cindy Rooks, and Cindy Stoeckl

Watercolors and illustrations: Amber Hansen

If you have any questions or comments or would like information on specialty products featured in this book, please contact: Chapelle Ltd., Inc., P.O. Box 9252 Ogden, UT 84409 • (801) 621-2777 • (801) 621-2788 (fax)

The written instructions, photographs, designs, patterns, and projects in this volume are intended for the personal use of the reader and may be reproduced for that purpose only. Any other use, especially commercial use, is forbidden under law without the written permission of the copyright holder. Every effort has been made to ensure that all the information in this book is accurate. However, due to differing conditions, tools, and individual skills, the publisher cannot be responsible for any injuries, losses, and other damages which may result from the use of the information in this book.

Library of Congress Cataloging-in-Publication Data

Hardy, Thomas, 1957–
    Great braids! : the new way to exciting hairstyles / Thomas Hardy.
        p. cm.
    Includes index.
    ISBN 0-8069-8615-8
    1. Braids (Hairdressing) 2. Hair-work. I. Title.
TT975.H37 1997
646.7'24--dc21   96-44347
                                                         CIP

10 9 8 7 6 5 4 3 2 1

Published by Sterling Publishing Company, Inc., 387 Park Avenue South, New York, NY 10016
© 1997 by Chapelle Limited
Distributed in Canada by Sterling Publishing c/o Canadian Manda group, One Atlantic Avenue, Suite 105, Toronto, Ontario, Canada M6K 3E7
Distributed in Great Britain and Europe by Cassell PLC, Wellington House, 125 Strand, London WC2R 0BB, England
Distributed in Australia by Capricorn Link (Australia) Pty Ltd., P.O. Box 6651, Baulkham Hills, Business Centre, NSW 2153, Australia
Printed in Hong Kong
All Rights Reserved

Sterling ISBN 0-8069-8615-8

ABOUT THE AUTHOR

Thomas Hardy's haircutting and design skills are known as some of the most progressive in the western United States. Performing extravaganzas and educational events from Canada to Bolivia have brought him national and international recognition. Magazines such as *Modern Salon, Teen Magazine, Passion,* and *Spanish Cosmopolitan* have featured his hairstyles and techniques.

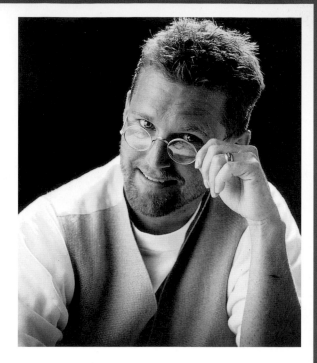

Thomas has received training from Vidal Sasson, Toni & Guy in London, and Horst & Friends in Minneapolis. Employing the knowledge he has gained, he has been recognized and featured in three educational videos for hair design. He has also done two major ad campaigns for hair care products manufacturer Image Laboratories. His hair designs have been featured in the Image Poster Collection. This same manufacturer awarded him the "Best of Show from an Image Artist." He has been praised not only for his cutting and design skills, but also for his talent in photographing his own work. His shoots have been located all over the world.

Thomas is currently an international artist for Graham Webb International, a hair care products manufacturer. He is owner and creative director of Rocky Mountain Hair, which was founded in 1981 in Ogden, Utah. On his team of stylists for this book is Sherrie Smith from St. Louis, Missouri. She created most of the braids featured. She is currently an Artistic Director for Graham Webb International.

FROM THE AUTHOR

Hair is one feature that can be quickly changed to create a mood or a feeling. In this book, I would like to share easy step-by-step instructions on how to create whatever mood is desired—from day styles to sporty looks to evening and glamour.

In all of my travels for hair shows, from Los Angeles to Rio de Janeiro, I ask the same question to my audiences, "When was the last time you locked yourself in the bathroom to practice with your own hair?" The answer is most definitely never! It is my wish to help you understand how easy it is to transform hair—whether it be your own or a friend's—into a work of art.

What is it that makes heads turn when a woman walks into a room? It is her ability to express her confidence; the state of knowing she looks her absolute best. Hair can play a major factor in how she feels about herself and the level of confidence she expresses. With tools such as this book and a little practice, incredibly beautiful hair is inevitable.

I was preparing this book while en route to New York for a hair show. A curious flight attendant, who had long beautiful hair, shared her own ideas of what she would like to see in an instructional hair styling book. We talked about the importance of having quick easy styles for women on the go in professional positions, as well as more elaborate styles that could be worn out on the town. Out of that conversation came this compilation of styles.

CONTENTS

Hair Care

Every Five to Seven Weeks:

• Trim ends to provide
  clean blunt lines.

Every Two Weeks:

• Apply deep conditioner to hair
  and sit in sauna or steam room.

Day to Day:

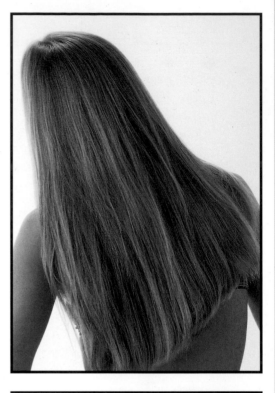

• Brush or pick hair before
  getting it wet.

• Avoid stretching or snapping hair
  which causes split ends.

• Cleanse with mild shampoo,
  massage scalp area, and rinse
  out shampoo from roots to ends.

• Apply conditioner to ends of hair
  and rinse out thoroughly.

• Rinse with cool water to close
  hair follicles and add shine.

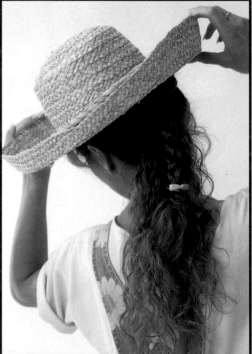

• Use large-tooth comb to detangle
  hair. Start with a small section of
  hair and comb out from the
  roots, a few inches at a time.

• Dry hair using low heat and
  styling products containing
  thermo protectors.

• Cover hair with a hat or tie
  it up with a visor while in the sun
  or tanning bed.

Styling Basics

There is nothing more beautiful than a head of hair that is properly cared for, cleansed, conditioned, and styled. Selecting the right products can be confusing because there are so many on the market. Consult a highly respected hairstylist in the local area who can recommend proper treatment.

Gels and mousses will be necessary in attaining this book's new hairstyles. These products allow the hairstyle to last longer. They also build body and create incredible shine. Be generous with mousse and apply evenly from roots to ends. It is important to keep heavy gels away from the scalp; they can weigh hair down and cause it to go flat.

Hair sprays are a great tool. They are important in maintaining a great hairstyle. Choose a working spray or a softer holding spray while building a new hairstyle. Add a firm holding spray to secure the hairstyle. For a touch of luster use a shining spray.

GADGETS & ACCESSORIES

Here are a few items used to create the hairstyles in this book and a few added just for fun. Remember that occasion, wardrobe, and hairstyle should influence the type of accessory selected.

Barrettes
These come in a variety of styles and sizes. They can be purchased at drug, department, and beauty supply stores.

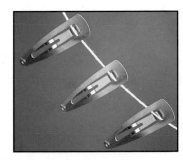
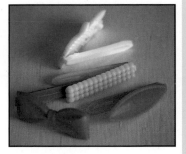

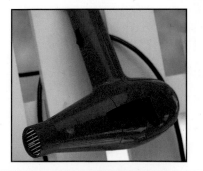

Blow Dryers
These come with different features. Some blow dryers come with attachments that direct air to one area. Others, with the push of a button, blow cool air onto desired curls, helping them keep their form. Blow dryers can be purchased at drug and beauty supply stores.

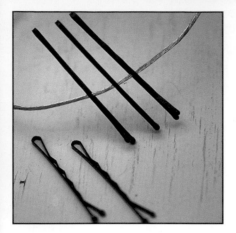

Bobby Pins

These come in dark and light colors. They are available in regular and large sizes. Bobby pins are used to secure hair tightly. They can be purchased at drug and beauty supply stores.

Brushes

These come in different types. A round brush is shown at the right. It is used with a blow dryer to curl the ends of hair under. A vent brush adds volume and air to roots. A paddle brush straightens hair. A denman brush is used to obtain smooth sleek hair. They can be purchased at beauty supply stores.

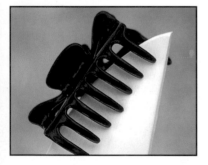

Butterfly Clips

These come in a variety of sizes, colors, and shapes. They can be used to hold sections of hair in place while working with other sections. They are also used in place of a barrette. Butterfly clips can be purchased at clothing and beauty supply stores.

Clips

These come in a variety of sizes and colors. They are used to hold sections of hair in place while working with other sections. Clips can be purchased at beauty supply stores.

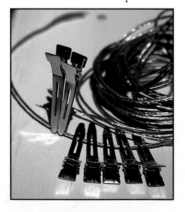

Small clips

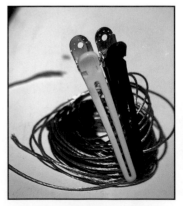

Large clips

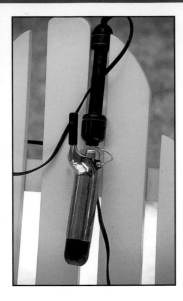

Curling Irons

These come with smooth or textured rods in a variety of sizes. Rod sizes range from ½" to 2" in diameter. The larger the rod the bigger the curl. Some models include a brush attachment. These attachments are used to get a smoother curl. Curling irons can be purchased at drug and beauty supply stores.

Curling Ropes

These are easily made at home from nylon rope which can be purchased at most hardware stores. Ropes are ¼" to ½" wide depending on desired curl size and are cut 14" in length. Ends are dipped in liquid plastic to prevent fraying.

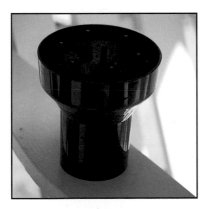

Diffusers

These are placed on the end of a blow dryer. They help to maintain curls and to prevent frizzy hair. Diffusers can be purchased at beauty supply stores.

Elastic Bands

These come in a variety of colors and sizes. They can be purchased at most drug or beauty supply stores. Common rubber bands should be avoided as they will pull the hair out.

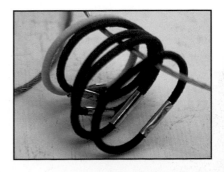

Hairpins

These come in different colors. They are used to tuck away loose unwanted hairs on a finished style or to place curls in a specific place. Hairpins can be purchased at drug and beauty supply stores.

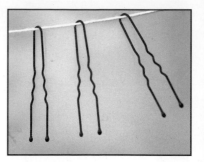

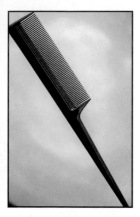

Long-Tailed Combs

These combs come with different size teeth. Large-tooth combs are best for detangling hair. Small-tooth combs add texture and smooth surface. They are used to tease hair and to fix bumpy spots in hairstyles. Long-tailed combs can be purchased at drug and beauty supply stores.

Picks

These come in different sizes. Full size picks work best on thick hair. Small or compact picks work best on finer hair. They can be purchased at drug and beauty supply stores.

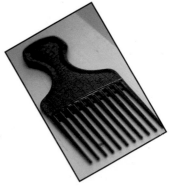

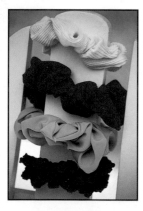

Scrunchies

These come in a variety of colors, fabrics, and sizes. They can be used to hide elastic bands and secure hair, but are mostly for decoration. They can be purchased at clothing, drug, and beauty supply stores.

Velcro Rollers

These come in different sizes. Use larger rollers for bigger curls. They are used for quick and easy curls. They can be purchased at drug and beauty supply stores.

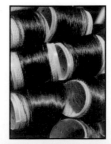

Barrette for Ribbons

Materials
- Plastic square with 10 holes and a metal barrette attached *
- Ribbon, 3 yards
- Sucker stick

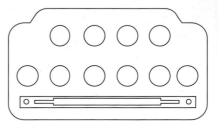

Instructions

1. Cut ribbon(s) into two or three equal lengths. (The more lengths used, the fuller the bow.)

2. Insert one length of ribbon through hole from clip side to front pulling to desired length.

3. Form a small loop on the clasp side and insert loop through next hole, pulling ribbon to front to desired size loop. (Use sucker stick to push ribbon through hole.)

4. Repeat in additional holes across row, pulling remaining ribbon through hole at other end to front.

5. Repeat steps 2–4 to thread the second row using the second length of ribbon. Ribbon ends are threaded through the same holes as first bow.

6. Trim ribbon ends, separate ribbon loops, shape and fluff to desired look.

To re-use barrette, simply remove ribbons by holding streamers at one end and pull until free.

* *Offray's Miracle Bow* was used for the project in this book.

Crochet Scrunchie

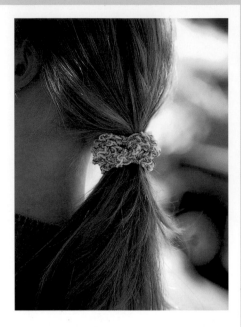

Materials
- Woven chainette, 20 yards each: aqua, iridescent
- Elastic ponytail ring or 9" of round elastic tied in a ring
- Crochet hook: size K

Instructions
Use 1 strand of each color of chainette together throughout.

1. Join chainettes with sl st around elastic ring.

2. Work around elastic ring. Ch 6, work sl st inserting hook through 6th ch from hook and under elastic ring. Repeat process 12 times.

3. Join with sl st in first ch of round, taking care not to twist chain, insert hook into first chain, yarn over and pull through chain and loop on hook.

4. Turn work on inside of ring with right side facing. Ch 6, work sl st inserting hook through 6th Ch from hook and under elastic ring between next 2 Ch loops. Repeat process 12 times.

5. Join with sl st in first ch of round, taking care not to twist chain, insert hook into first chain or round. Fasten off.

sl st = slip stitch
ch = chain(s)

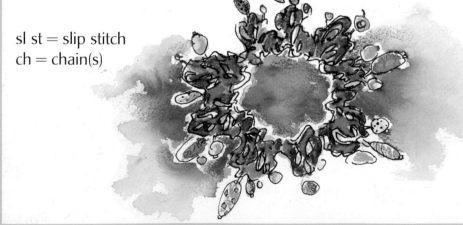

Off-Centered Rose

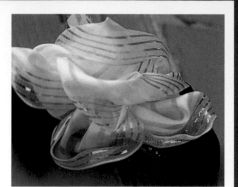

Materials
- Ribbon, 1½" wide: 18" taffeta, 12" sheer, 18" sheer
- Craft barrette
- Disappearing white-ink fabric marker
- Needle
- Thread
- Hot glue gun and glue sticks

Instructions

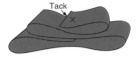

1. Loosely fold 18" taffeta back on itself four times as shown in diagram forming a stacked ribbon.

2. Tack ribbons together at center with thread to form a bow.

3. Make a multiple-petaled flower with 12" taffeta. See step 3 of Multi-Petaled Flower (page 16). Set aside.

4. Make a gathered rose with 18" sheer ribbon. See Gathered Rose (page15). Pull rose slightly off center. Secure rose below center bow with thread. Knot to secure.

5. Place multiple-petaled flower above rose and secure with hot glue. Secure arrangement to barrette with hot glue.

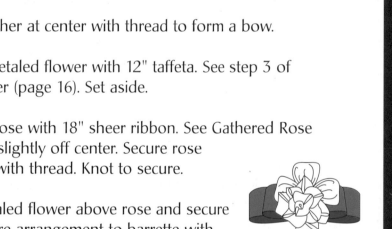

Ponytail Rose

Materials
- Ribbon, 1½" wide: 24" taffeta
- Craft barrette for ponytails
- Needle
- Thread
- Hot glue gun and glue sticks

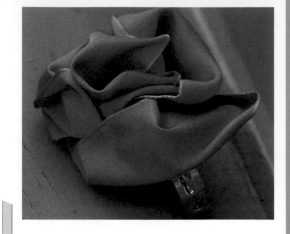

Instructions

1. Start at center of taffeta and fold into an "L" shape to the right at a right angle.

2. Fold and press horizontal leg to the back so it extends to the left.

3. Fold vertical leg to back so it extends downward.

4. Fold horizontal leg to back so it extends to right. Continue folding each leg in turn, always back, alternating directions so the previous fold is secured.

5. When taffeta ends are reached, hold the last fold and its leg firmly between thumb and forefinger. Let folded section release itself.

pull

6. Pull the other leg through the folds. Tack the base of rose at center. Knot to secure.

hold

7. Secure arrangement to barrette with hot glue.

Tack at base

Velvet Hair Stick

Materials
- Velvet tubing: 30" long, black
- Pointed stick: 5½" long (chopstick)
- Bead for end of stick: black
- Jewel pin: to fit hole in bead
- Acrylic paint: copper, bronze
- Paint brush
- Hot glue gun and glue sticks

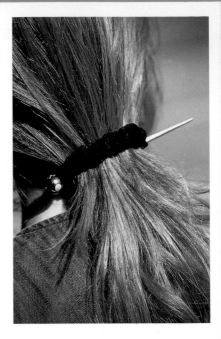

Instructions
1. Take one end of velvet tubing and loop over 1½".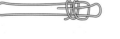

2. Glue loop in place. Allow to dry.

3. Make another loop 4¾" from first glued loop.

4. Pinch and hold second loop while wrapping tubing from one end to the other. Continue wrapping until opposite end is reached.

5. Tuck end back into wrapped section. Secure with hot glue.

6. Mix a small amount of copper in with the bronze. Paint stick and allow to dry. Paint bead if desired.

7. Insert jewelry pin through bead and push it through the square end of stick.

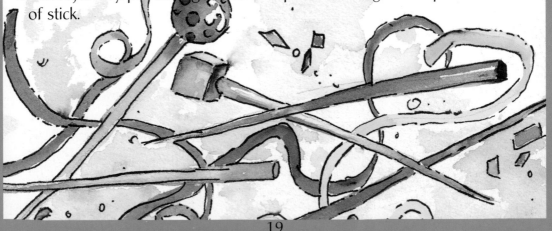

HAND POSITIONS FOR BRAIDING

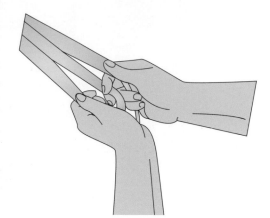

1. Divide hair into three even sections. Hold outer sections with thumbs and index fingers as shown. Hold center section between middle finger and index finger of right hand.

2. Turn right palm toward the ground, crossing right section over center section. Move center section over to right hand, holding it between middle finger and index finger of right hand.

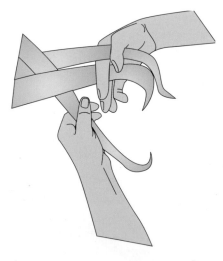

3. Turn left palm toward the ground, crossing left section over center section. Move center section over to left hand, holding it between middle finger and index finger of left hand. Repeat steps 2 and 3 until all hair is braided. Secure with an elastic band.

HAND POSITIONS FOR BRAIDING OWN HAIR

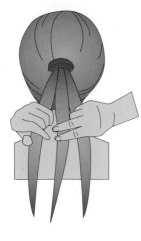

1. Start with hair in a ponytail or desired position on head. Divide hair into three even sections. Hold right section in right hand with index and middle finger extended. Grab center section with extended fingers and position it between middle and ring finger.

2. Cross right section over center section, securing with middle finger of left hand. Pull center section to the right.

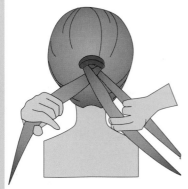

3. Cross left section over this new center section, securing hair with middle finger of right hand. Pull center section to the left.

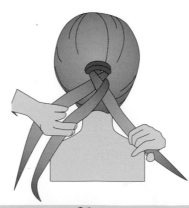

4. Repeat steps 2 and 3 until all hair is braided. Secure with an elastic band.

OPEN FILE SYSTEM

The Open File System of braiding is a relaxing way to hold the hands while braiding other people's hair. This technique offers the following advantages over other methods of braiding:

- More control over the braid
- Easier straightening and tightening of the hair
- Less tension on the hands
- Easier means of correcting errors

Divided sections of hair are placed into "files." A file is the area between two fingers. One hand needs to be completely filed, or have strands of hair in each indicated area on the hand, before moving files to the other hand. Numbering for the files always begins from the pinky side and counts off toward the thumb. The basic rules for the Open File System are:

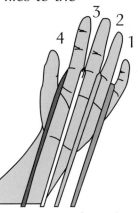

- Keep palm open and relaxed at all times.
- Rest knuckle of middle finger against the scalp.
- Start with files on the left hand.

The Open File System can be used on any braid. The secret is to adapt the hands to the type of braid desired. This book shows how to use the Open File System for the Basic Braid, French Braid, Inside-Out Braid, and Four Strand Braid.

The Open File System will be easier for those who have never braided. For those who have used other methods of braiding, there may be a tendency to switch from one method to another, undoing the braid. Do not get frustrated. Keep practicing, with the palms open and relaxed. Beginner and expert braiders will love this system once it is mastered.

BRAIDS

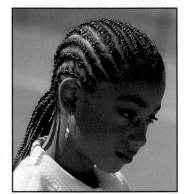

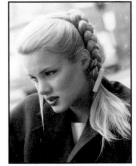

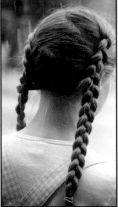

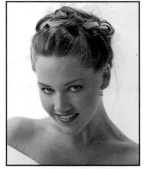

All
the braids in this book
will work for hair that is shoulder
length or longer. People with shorter hair
can create these braids in different sections of
their hair. Braiding might be easy for some and a
struggle for others. The key to creating a new
hairstyle is practice. It takes a few tries to get it right.
If a hairstyle has a few bumps or gaps after
braiding, fix them with a long–tailed comb. Push
the comb under the top layer of hair where
the problem has occurred. Move the
comb down through the hair and
over the bump or gap.

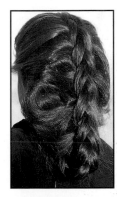

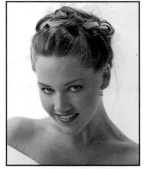

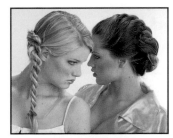

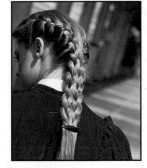

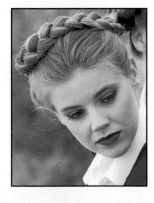

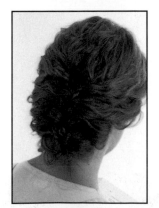

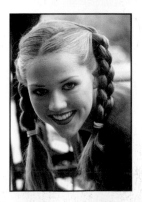

BASIC BRAID

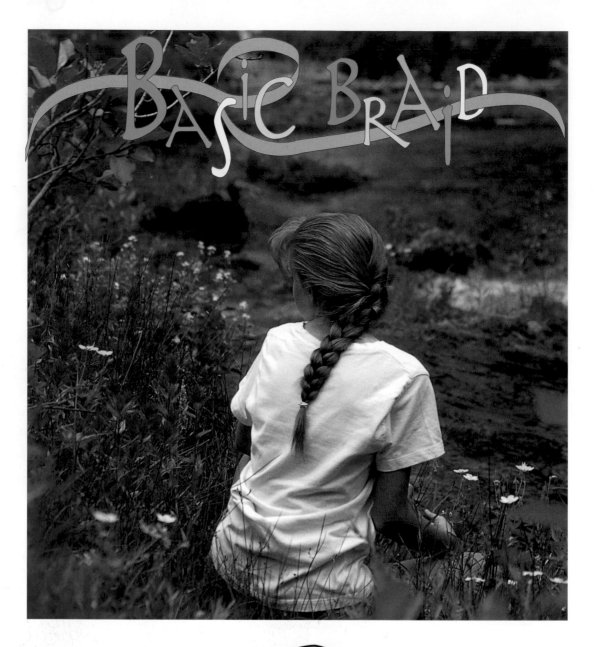

The Basic Braid is the root of all braids. It can be started from a ponytail or any position on head.

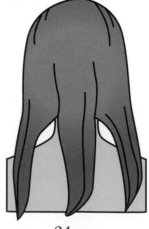

1 Divide hair into three even sections.

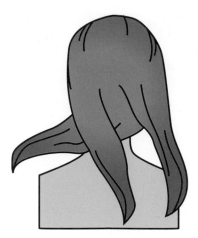

2 Cross left section over center section, making it the new center section.

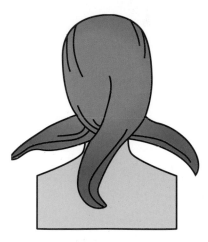

3 Cross right section over center, making it the new center section.

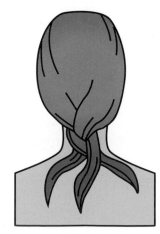

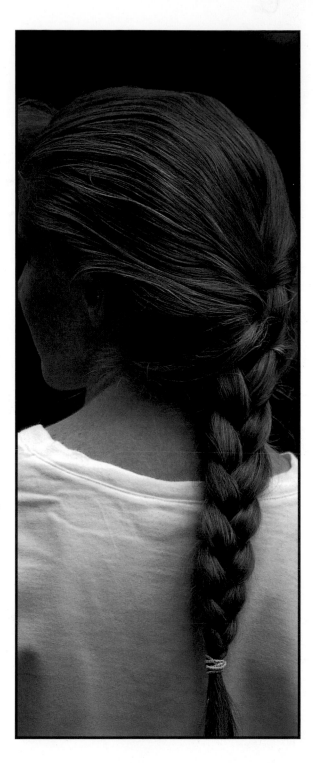

4 Repeat steps 2 and 3 until braid reaches desired length. Secure with an elastic band.

Basic Braid Open File System

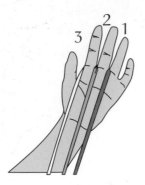

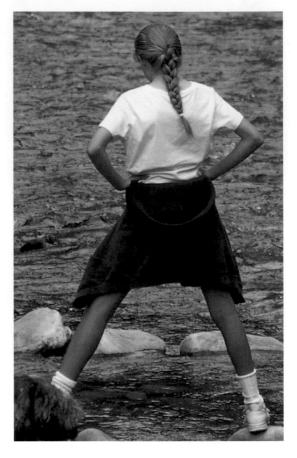

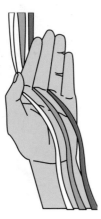

1
Divide hair into three even sections. Place the sections of hair into files #1, #2, and #3 of left hand.

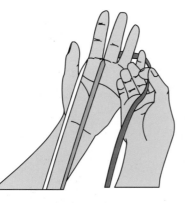

2
Pick up hair in file #1 with index finger and thumb of right hand, moving hair to right hand.

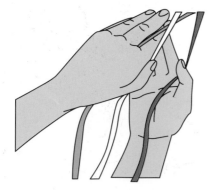

3
Switch files #2 and #3 by turning left palm toward the ground. Insert middle finger of right hand between files #2 and #3, moving hair to right hand.

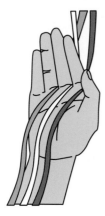

4

Right hand is now filed. Tighten and straighten hair as needed.

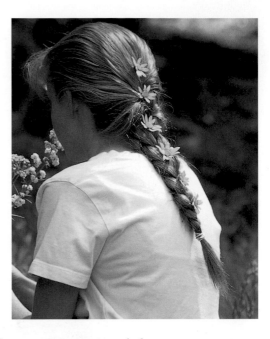

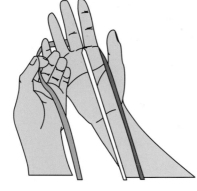

5

Repeat the same process on left hand. Pick up hair from file #1 with index finger and thumb of left hand, moving hair to left hand.

6

Switch files #2 and #3 by turning right palm toward the ground. Insert middle finger of left hand between files #2 and #3, moving hair to left hand.

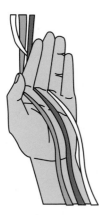

7

Left hand is now filed. Tighten and straighten hair as needed. Repeat steps 2–6 until all hair is braided. Secure with an elastic band.

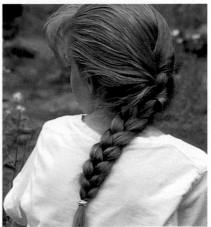

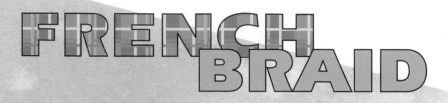

FRENCH BRAID

The French Braid is like the Basic Braid (page 24), except that hair is gradually added into the three sections.

Helpful Hints

• Gather strands of hair 2-3" wide.

• Tug down on hair to tighten.

• Add narrow strands of hair for a more formal braid.

• Add wide strands of hair for a casual braid.

• Be consistent in strand size.

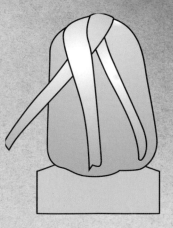

1. Gather a section of hair at top of head and divide gathered hair into three even sections. Cross right section over center section. Cross left section over new center section making one basic braid.

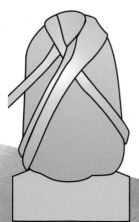

2. Pull a small strand of hair from right side of head and add it to right section of braid. Cross right section over center section. Pull center section all the way to the right.

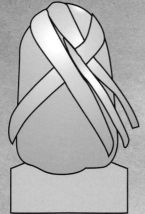

3. Pull a small strand of hair from left side of head and add it to left section of braid. Cross left section over center section. Pull center section all the way to left.

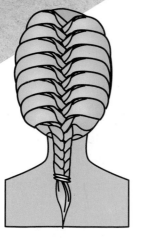

4. Repeat steps 2 and 3 until all hair has been added into the braid. Continue with the Basic Braid (page 24). Secure with an elastic band.

French Braid
Open File System

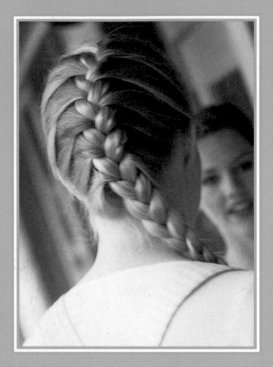

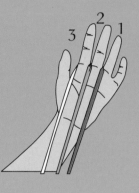

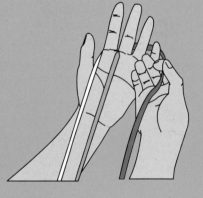

1
Divide hair into three even sections. Place sections of hair into files #1, #2, and #3 of left hand.

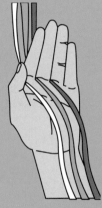

2
Pull a small strand of hair back from the right side of head and place in file #1. Pick up hair in file #1 with index finger and thumb of right hand, moving hair to right hand.

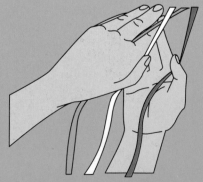

3
Switch files #2 and #3 by turning left palm toward the ground. Insert middle finger of right hand between files #2 and #3, moving hair to right hand.

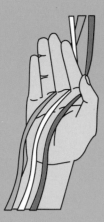

4

Right hand is now filed. Tighten and straighten hair as needed.

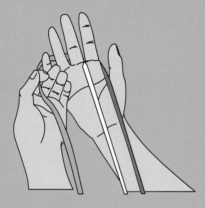

This style is a French Braid that has been tucked. See Tucked Braids (page 68).

5

Repeat the same process on left hand. Pull a small strand of hair back from the left side of head and place in file #1. Pick up hair from file #1 with index finger and thumb of left hand, moving hair to left hand.

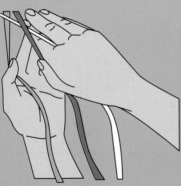

6

Switch files #2 and #3 by turning right palm toward the ground. Insert middle finger of left hand between files #2 and #3, moving hair to left hand.

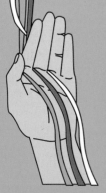

7

Left hand is now filed. Tighten and straighten hair as needed. Repeat steps 2-6 until all hair is braided. Finish with the Basic Braid (page 26). Secure with an elastic band.

inside-out braid

This braid can be used anywhere a French Braid is used. The strands on this braid always cross **under** the center section.

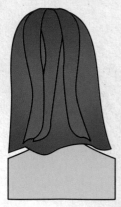

1. Gather a section of hair at top of head and divide gathered hair into three even sections.

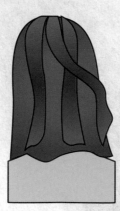

2. Cross right section under center section. Pull center section all the way to the right.

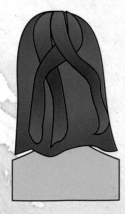

3. Pull left section under new center section. Pull center section all the way to the right.

This style of the Inside-Out Braid is draped. See Draped Braids (page 69).

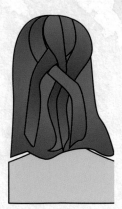

4. Pull a small strand from right side of head and add it to right section. Cross right section under center section. Pull center section all the way to the right.

5. Pull a small strand of hair from left side of head and add it to left section. Cross left section under center section. Pull center section all the way to the left.

6. Repeat steps 3-5 until all hair has been added into braid. Proceed with the Basic Braid (page 24), continuing to cross hair under center section. Secure with an elastic band.

Inside-Out Braid Open File System

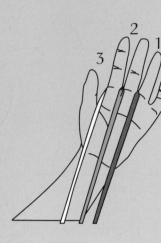

1 Gather hair at top of head. Divide gathered hair into three even sections. Place the three sections of hair into files #1, #2, and #3 of left hand.

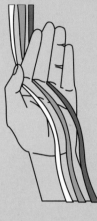

2 Pull a small strand of hair from right side of the head and add it to file #1.

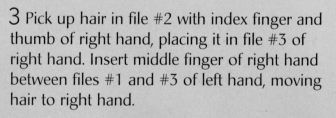

3 Pick up hair in file #2 with index finger and thumb of right hand, placing it in file #3 of right hand. Insert middle finger of right hand between files #1 and #3 of left hand, moving hair to right hand.

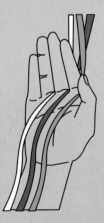

4 Right hand is now filed. Tighten and straighten hair as needed. Pull a small section of hair from left side of the head and add it to file #1.

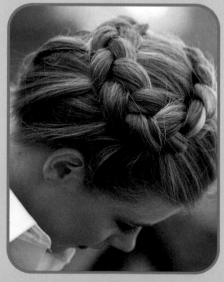

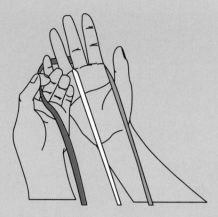

5 Pick up hair in file #2 with index finger and thumb of left hand, placing it in file #3 of left hand. Insert middle finger of right hand between files #1 and #3 of left hand, moving hair to left hand.

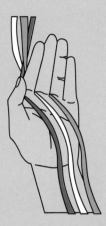

6 Left hand is now filed. Straighten and tighten hair as needed. Repeat steps 2-5 until all hair has been added. Finish with the Basic Braid (page 26). Secure with an elastic band.

This style is the Inside-Out Braid on each side of the head. The zigzag parts are not necessary for this look. Any part desired will work fine.

The style pictured on the opposite page is the Inside-Out Braid braided around the head. See The Bride (page 60) for instructions.

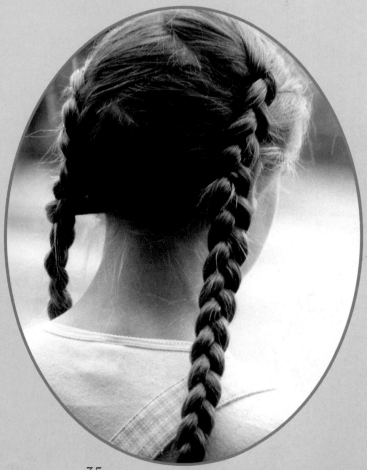

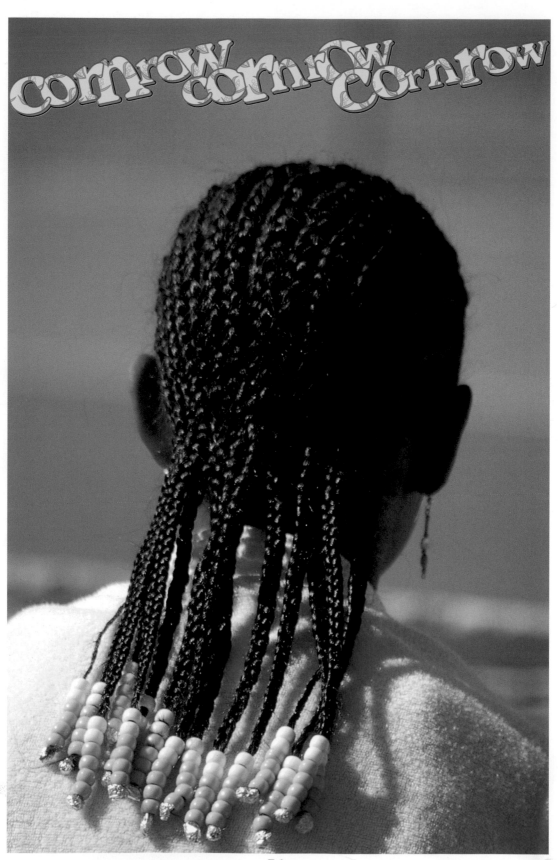

Cornrows are many narrow French Braids (page 28) or Inside-Out Braids (page 32) running parallel to each other positioned along the scalp.

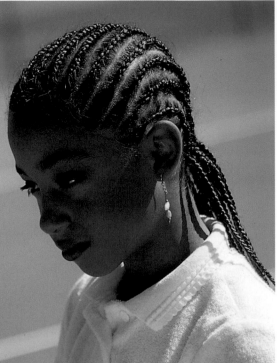

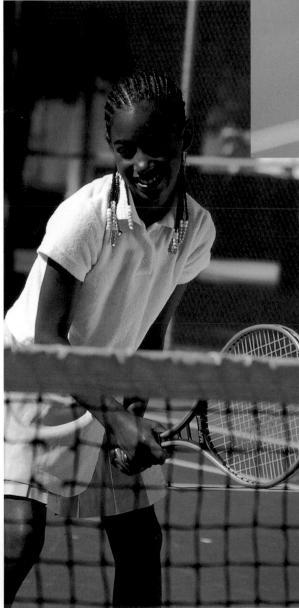

Helpful Hints

• Try to pick up the same amount of hair each time.

• Secure ends by wrapping and knotting with thread.

• Make clear parts between braids for comfort and a clean look.

• Avoid braiding hair into the wrong section as it may break hair and pull on the scalp.

• Avoid placing heavy beads on fragile hair.

• Use versatile colors of beads as braids can stay in hair for several days.

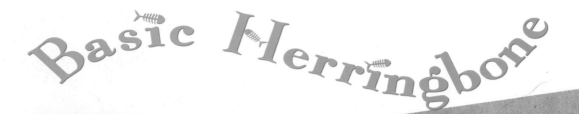

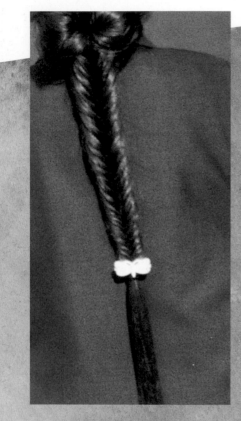

Helpful Hints

• Pull strands tight.

• Use wide strands for an informal look.

• Use narrow strands for a formal look.

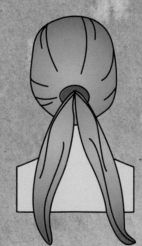

1

Gather hair at desired position on head or in a ponytail. Secure with an elastic band. Divide ponytail into two sections.

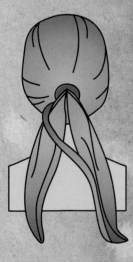

2

Pull a narrow strand of hair out from under left section and cross it over to join right section.

3

Pull a narrow strand of hair out from under right section and cross it over to join left section.

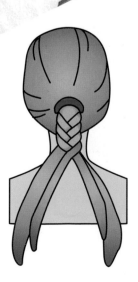

4

Repeat steps 2 and 3, always pulling a new strand from under gathered hair. Secure with an elastic band or barrette.

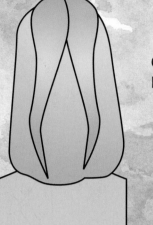

1

Gather a section of hair at the top of head.
Divide the gathered section in half.

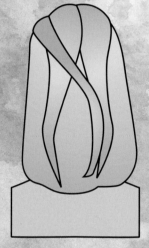

2

Pull a narrow strand of
hair from left side of
head. Cross it over left
section and add it to the
right section.

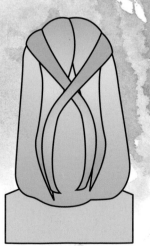

3

Pull a narrow strand of hair from right side of head.
Cross it over right section and add it to left section.

40

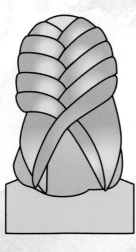

4

Repeat steps 2 and 3 until all hair has been gathered into the braid. Secure with an elastic band or barrette, or continue with the Basic Herringbone (page 38).

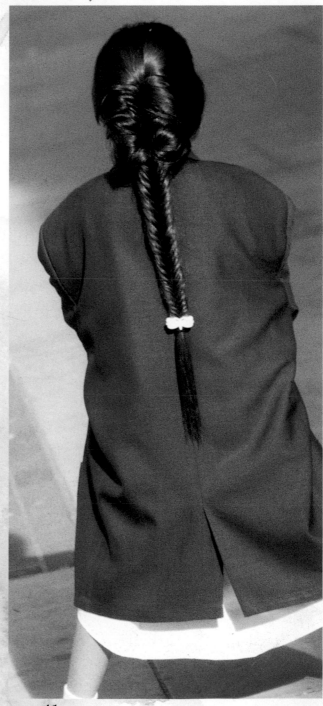

upside-down BRAID

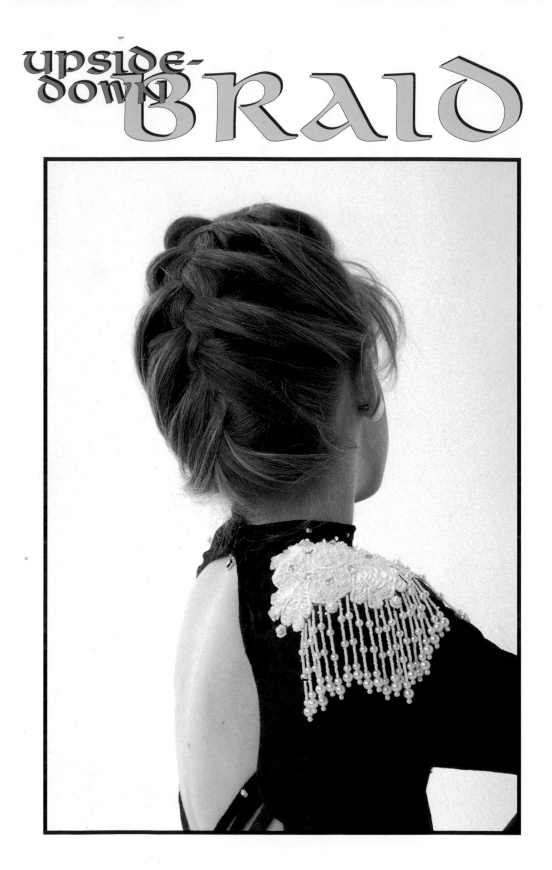

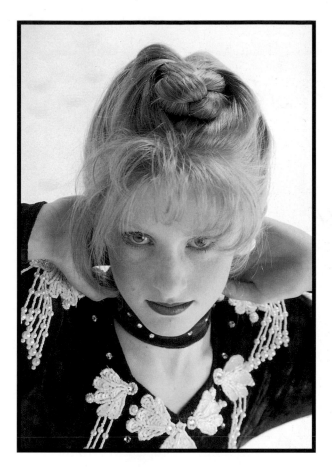

This style is created by following steps 1 and 2 and continuing the French Braid (page 28) until all hair is added. Finish with the Basic Braid (page 24). Tuck tail back into French Braid and secure with bobby pins.

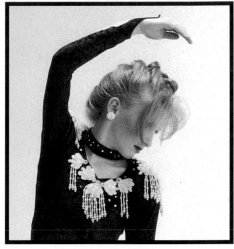

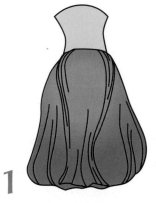

1

Hang head down and comb all hair toward the ground. Gather a wide section of hair from nape of neck.

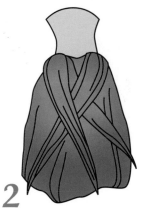

2

Start the French Braid (page 28), working from neck down to crown of head.

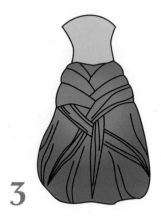

3

Stop after four to five rounds of braiding.

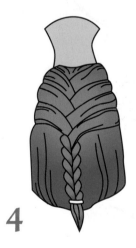

4

Make the Basic Braid (page 24) without picking up additional hair to make sure French Braid does not come undone. Secure with an elastic band.

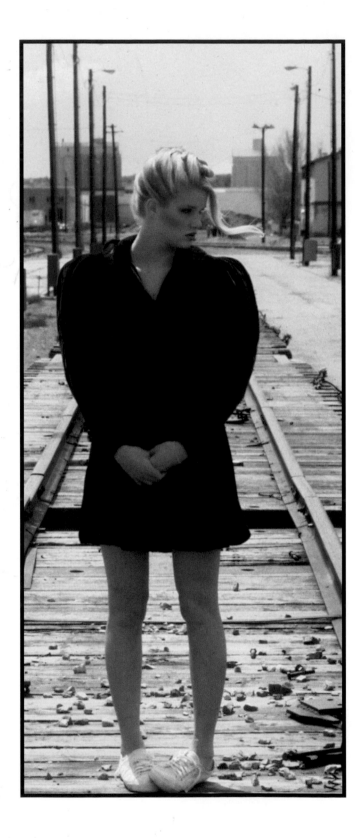

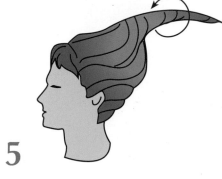

5

Put head up straight and gather unbraided hair together with braided section high on head. Twist gathered hair in one direction.

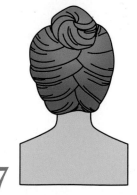

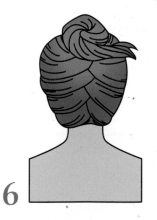

6

Continue twisting all hair and coil it around itself. Tuck ends under.

7

Secure with bobby pins.

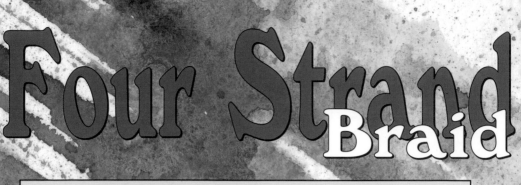

Four Strand Braid

The Four Strand Braid is a thick dimensional braid. It is made by using the Open File System (page 22).

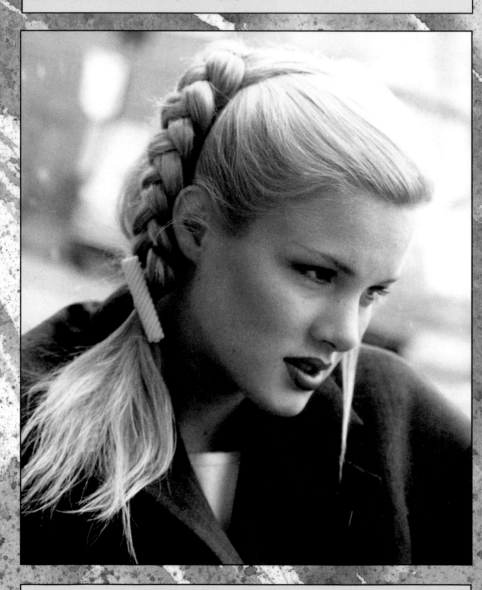

This style is created by starting the Four Strand Braid from a ponytail. It is secured with a barrette.

1. Divide hair into four even sections. Place four sections of hair into files #1, #2, #3, and #4 of left hand.

2. Pick up hair in file #3 with index finger and thumb of right hand, placing it in file #4 of right hand.

3. Grab file #1 with middle and index finger of right hand and place it in file #3 of right hand.

This style is created by starting the Four Strand Braid from pigtails. Hair is parted in a zigzag to the right.

4. Switch files #2 and #4 by turning palm of left hand toward the ground. Insert ring finger of right hand through files #2 and #4, moving hair to right hand.

5. Right hand is now filed. Tighten and straighten hair as needed.

6. Repeat the same process on left hand. Pick up hair in file #3 with index finger and thumb of left hand, placing it in file #4 of left hand.

7. Grab file #1 with middle and index finger of left hand and place it in file #3 of left hand.

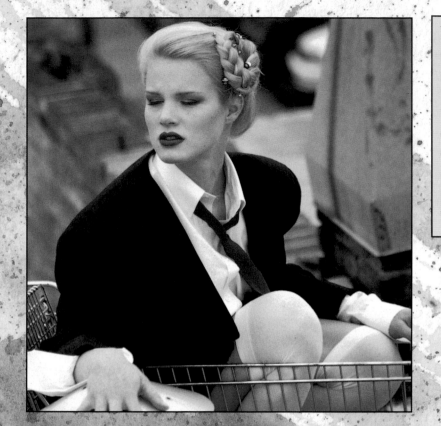

This style is created by placing one Four Strand Braid above the ear on each side of the head. The braid is looped up and secured with hairpins.

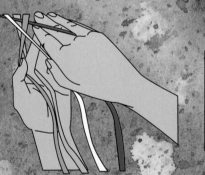

8. Switch files #2 and #4 by turning palm of right hand toward the ground. Insert ring finger of left hand through files #2 and #4, moving hair to left hand.

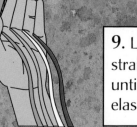

9. Left hand is now filed. Tighten and straighten hair as needed. Repeat steps 2-8 until all hair is braided. Secure with an elastic band.

French Four Strand Braid

The French Four Strand Braid is a cross between the French Braid (page 30) and the Four Strand Braid (page 46). It is made by using the Open File System (page 22).

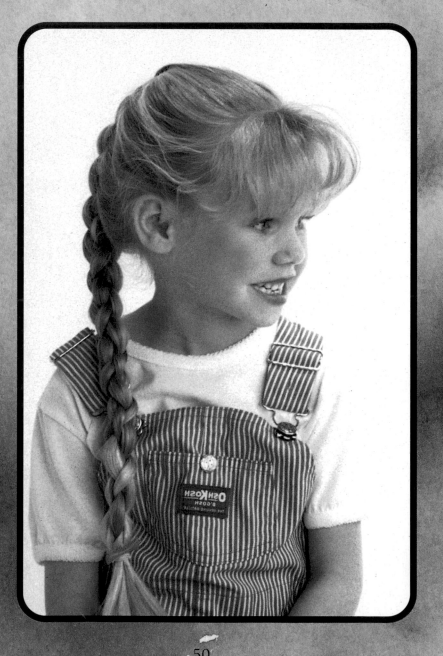

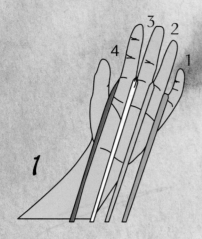

Divide hair into four even sections.
Place four sections of hair into
files of left hand.

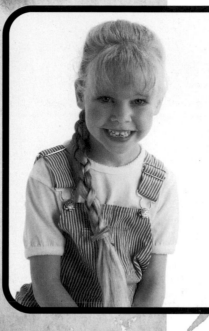

Pull a small strand of hair from right
side of head and add it to file #1. Pick
up hair in file #3 with index finger and
thumb of right hand and place it in file
#4 of right hand.

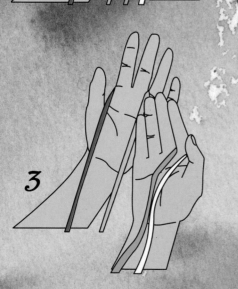

Grab file #1 with middle and index
finger of right hand and place it in
file #3 of right hand.

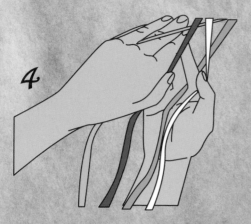

4

Switch files #2 and #4 by turning palm of left hand toward the ground. Insert ring finger of right hand through files #2 and #4, moving hair to right hand.

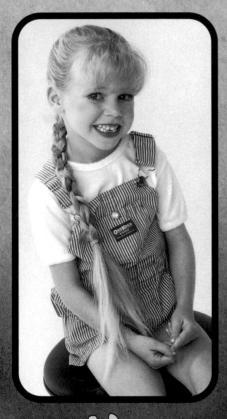

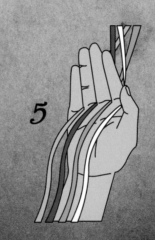

5 Right hand is now filed. Tighten and straighten hair as needed.

6

Repeat the same process on left hand. Pull a small strand of hair from the left side of head and add it to file #1. Pick up hair in file #3 with index finger and thumb of left hand and place it in file #4 of left hand.

52

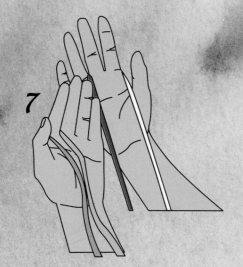

7 Grab file #1 with middle and index finger of left hand, placing it in file #3 of left hand.

8 Switch files #2 and #4 by turning palm of right hand toward the ground. Insert ring finger of left hand through files #2 and #4, moving hair to left hand.

9 Left hand is now filed. Tighten and straighten hair as needed. Repeat steps 2-8 until all hair has been added. Finish with the Four Strand Braid (page 46). Secure with an elastic band.

Rope Braid

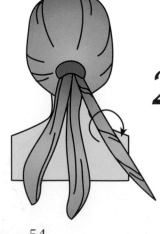

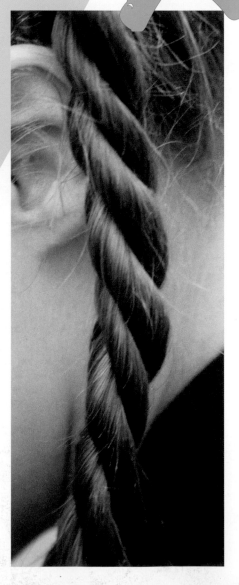

Helpful Hints

• Try braiding with slightly damp hair.

• Twist hair to the right each time.

• Ponytail can be secured with an elastic band, if desired.

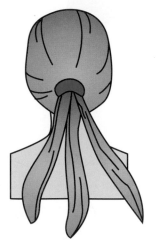

1 Gather hair in desired position on head or in a ponytail. Divide hair into three even sections.

2 Twist right section to right several times.

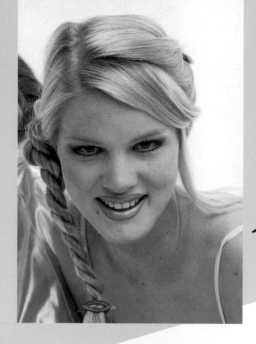

3 Cross right section over left and center sections.

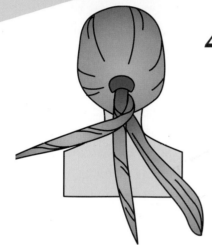

4 Repeat steps 2 and 3 until all desired hair is roped. Secure with an elastic band.

Remember: placement and parting make a difference in the outcome of a braid.

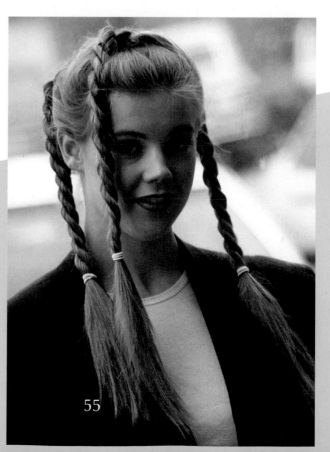

French rope

The French Rope is a combination of the Rope Braid (page 54) and French Braid (page 28).

This style is created by dividing hair in half down the back. French Rope one section until all hair is added. Repeat process on other section. Both sections are combined with the Rope Braid (page 54). Secure with an elastic band.

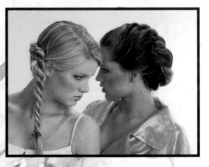

1

Gather a handful of hair at top of head and divide into three even sections. Cross right section over center section and then left section over the center section as if starting the Basic Braid (page 24).

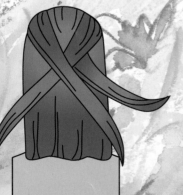

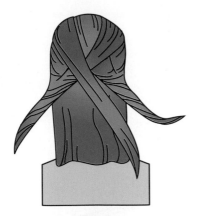

2

Pull a small strand of hair from right side of head and add to right section. Twist it to the right a few times. Pull a small strand of hair from left side of head and add to left section. Twist to the right a few times.

3

Cross right section over left and center sections. Repeat steps 2 and 3 until all hair has been roped. (If the braid does not look like those pictured in the beginning, do not worry. The braid begins taking the form of a rope about halfway down the head.)

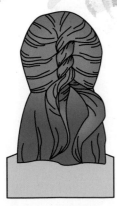

4

Continue to rope remaining hair in the Rope Braid (page 54). Secure with an elastic band.

CLIPPED
BRAIDS

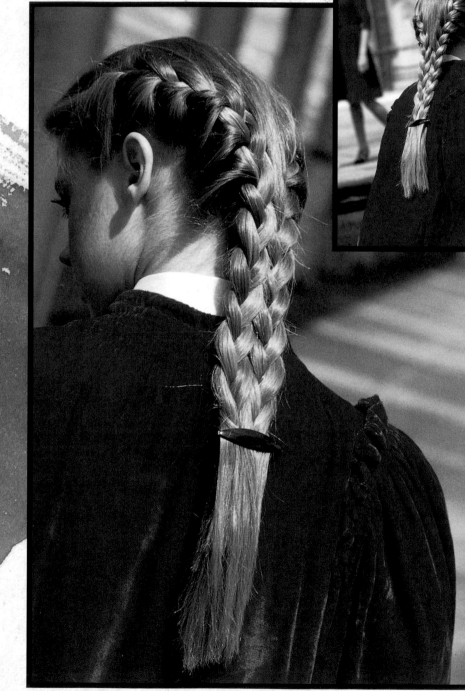

This style is created with two Inside-Out Braids (page 32 or page 34), two Basic Braids (page 24 or page 26), bobby pins, and a barrette. The Inside-Out Braid can be substituted with the French Braid.

1 Divide hair into two sections. Clip right side of hair or place over the shoulder to keep it out of the way. Make an Inside-Out Braid on left section of hair until all hair has been added. Finish with the Basic Braid. Secure with an elastic band.

2 Make an Inside-Out Braid on right section of hair until all hair has been added. Finish with the Basic Braid. Secure with an elastic band.

3 Clip the two braids together with two bobby pins behind braids at nape of neck. Cover elastic bands with a barrette.

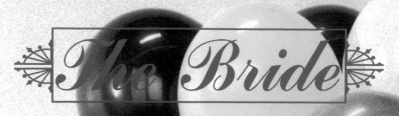

The Bride

This style is created by using an Inside-Out Braid (page 34) with tulle. The tulle is placed in each file and braided along with hair. The amount of tulle needed is double the hair length. Ribbon can be used instead of tulle.

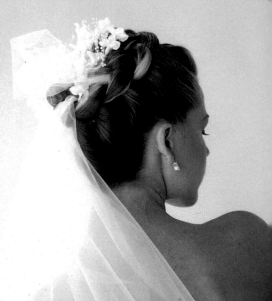

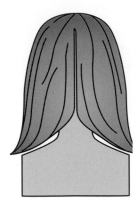

1 Divide hair in half down the back. Start on right side of head in the center. Begin braiding an Inside–Out Braid (page 32 or page 34).

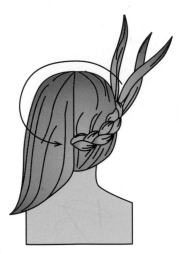

2 Keep braiding hair around head in a circle.

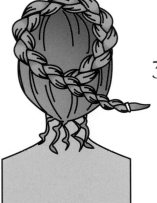

3 After all hair has been added, finish with the Basic Braid (page 24 or page 26). Secure with an elastic band.

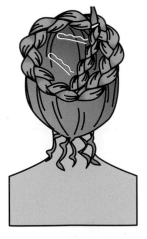

4 Tuck tail of braid into side of crown. Secure with hairpins as needed.

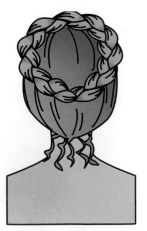

5 Curl pieces of hair that have fallen out with a curling iron.

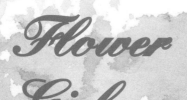

Flower Girl Braid

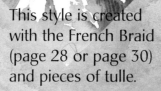

This style is created
with the French Braid
(page 28 or page 30)
and pieces of tulle.

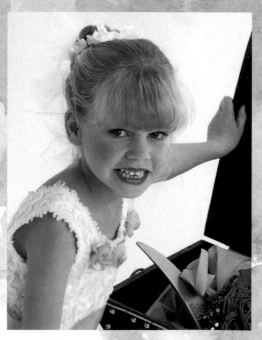

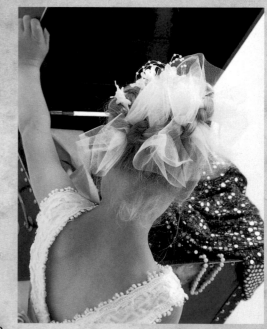

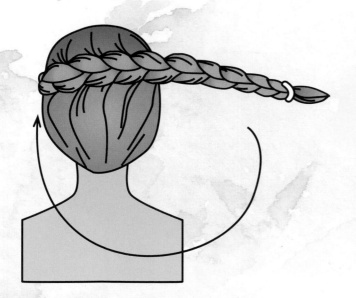

one

Begin a French Braid (page 28 or page 30) above left ear. Braid straight across center of head as shown in diagram. After all hair has been added, finish with the Basic Braid (page 24 or page 26) adding tulle as desired. Secure with an elastic band.

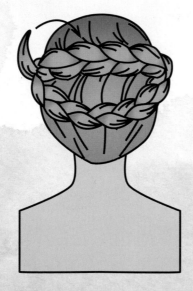

two

Wrap tail of braid to left and below French Braid. Tuck end into braid. Secure with bobby pins as needed.

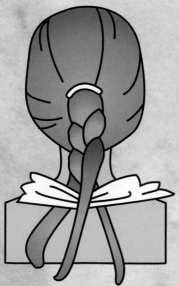

adding tulle to braids

Cut tulle into pieces 5" in length. Place tulle in the Basic Braid every fourth round underneath center section as shown.

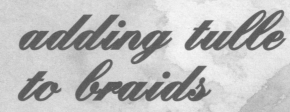

Wrapped Crown Braid

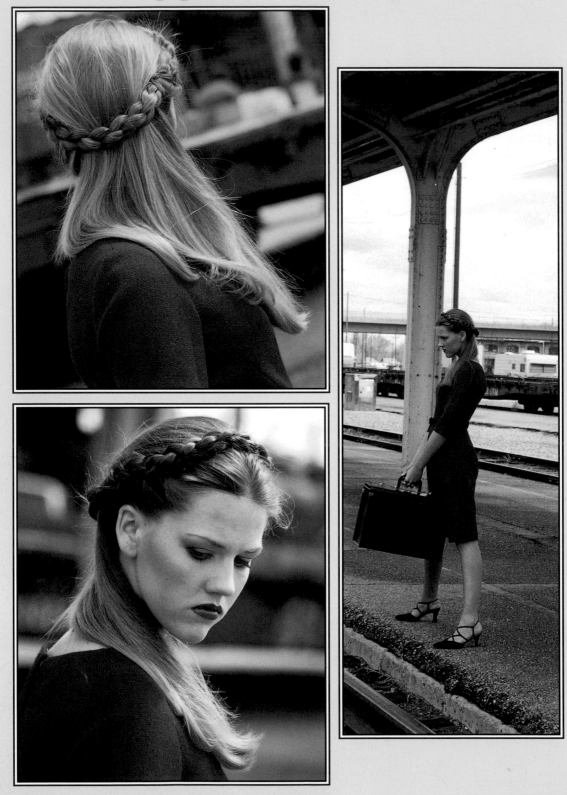

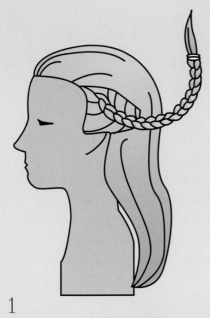

1

Take a 3" section above ear on left side of head. Start the French Four Strand Braid (page 50) toward back of head, stopping after three to five rounds. Continue to braid section with the Four Strand Braid (page 46). Secure with an elastic band.

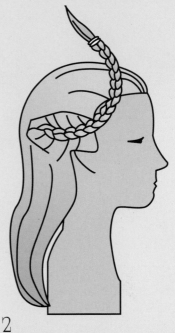

2

Take a 3" section above ear on right side of head. Start the French Four Strand Braid (page 50) toward face, stopping after three to five rounds. Continue to braid section with the Four Strand Braid (page 46). Secure with an elastic band.

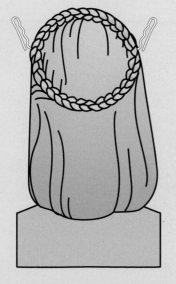

3

Wrap left braid around back of head. Secure braid in place with a hairpin. Wrap right around front of head, creating a crown. Tuck braid ends into crown. Secure with hairpins as needed.

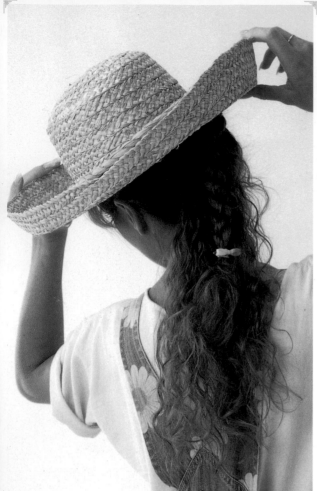

Scrunched Four Strand Braid

This style is created with two Four Strand Braids (page 46) that meet and form one braid in back. Hair has been prepared before braiding by using gel or mousse and scrunching under a diffuser.

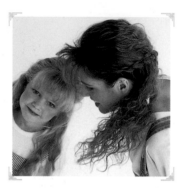

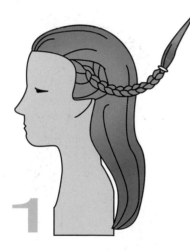

1 Take a 3" section of hair from behind left ear. Braid ¾ of section into the Four Strand Braid (page 46). Secure with a clip or an elastic band.

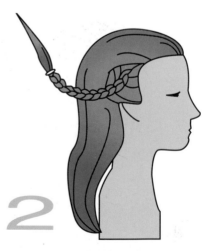

2 Take a 3" section of hair from above right ear. Braid ¾ of section into the Four Strand Braid (page 46). Secure with a clip or an elastic band.

66

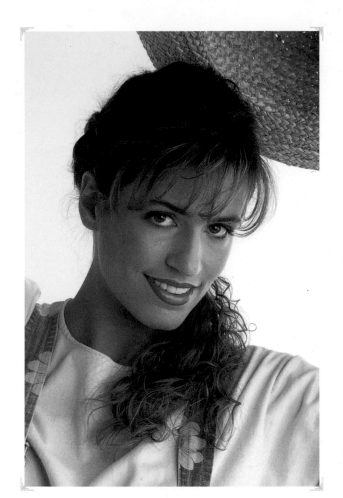

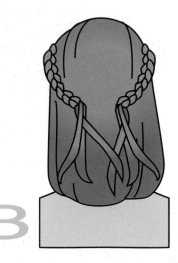

3 Wrap braids around back of head. Place two braids side by side, making sure braids are the same length.

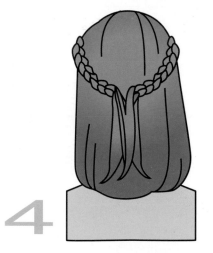

4 Remove clips or elastic bands. Combine unbraided sections of hair and continue with the Four Strand Braid (page 46).

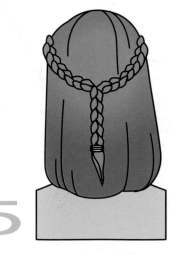

5 Secure braid with an elastic band or a barrette.

Tucked Braids

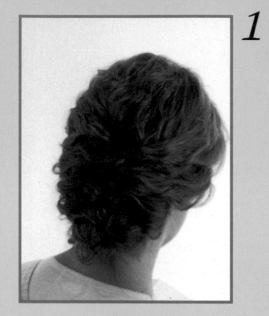

1 Braid hair in any braid desired. Leave braid a little loose toward bottom near neck by pulling the hands away from head as the last few sections of hair are being braided.

2 Carefully divide hair under braid, creating an opening and tuck tail of braid up into it. Secure with hairpins or bobby pins.

This
style is
created by
pulling back
both sides of
hair, leaving the
hair in the middle
alone. Keep braid loose.

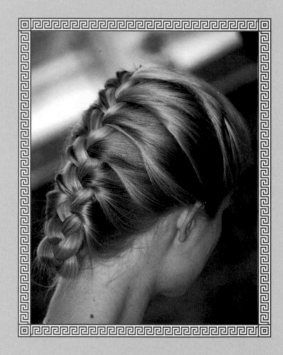

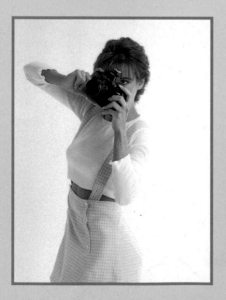

This
style is
created by
starting the braid
higher on the head
and pulling strands tightly.

This style is an Upside-Down Braid (page 42). Tucks can be done on any braid.

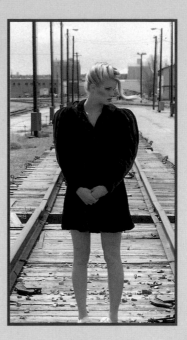

Draped Braids

Draping can be used on the French Braid (page 28 or page 30), Inside-Out Braid (page 32 or page 34), and Four Strand Braid (page 46). The key is to keep the hands away from the head while braiding.

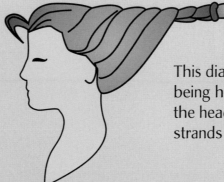

This diagram shows hair being held straight out from the head with very narrow strands being added.

Hold hands at an angle away from head. The size of the angle in which the hands are held will determine the final outcome of the braid. The French Herringbone (page 40) does not need to be draped. It already has a natural drape.

Beyond Braids

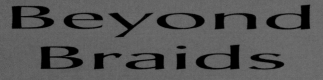

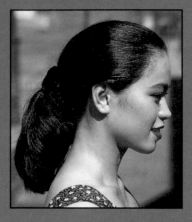

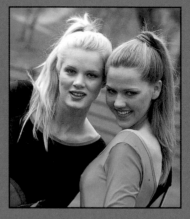

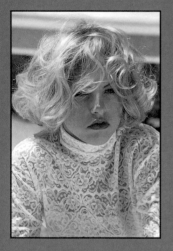

The styles in this section can be adapted to work with most hair lengths. When starting a new hairstyle always brush or comb hair to get rid of tangles and snarls. It may take two or three practice tries to get the desired style.

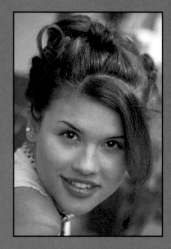

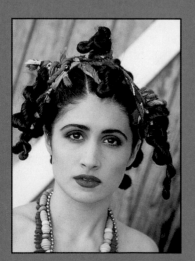

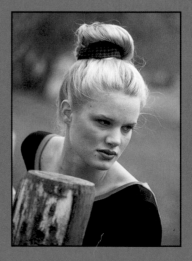

Curls Curls Curls Curls

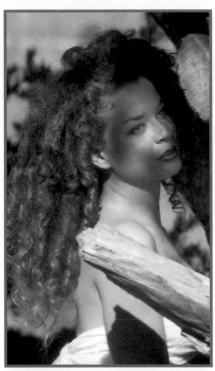

1 Saturate hair with mousse when damp. Use a blow dryer to dry completely.

2 Take 1" square parting. Use a ¾" curling iron and run hair from one end of curling iron to the other in a spiralling motion. Continue until all hair is curled.

3 Spray all curls with a light hair spray.

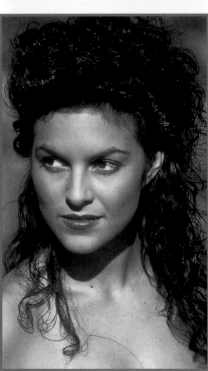

1 Apply a light sculpting gel to hair when damp. Use small rags as hair rollers and roll hair from ends to roots. Knot rags to secure. Continue until all hair is rolled.

2 Place hair under a dryer for 13 minutes or dry with a blow dryer for 15 minutes.

3 Remove rags and break curls apart with fingers. Spray all curls with a light hair spray. Pull sides up to top of head and secure with large barrette.

Velcro Rollers

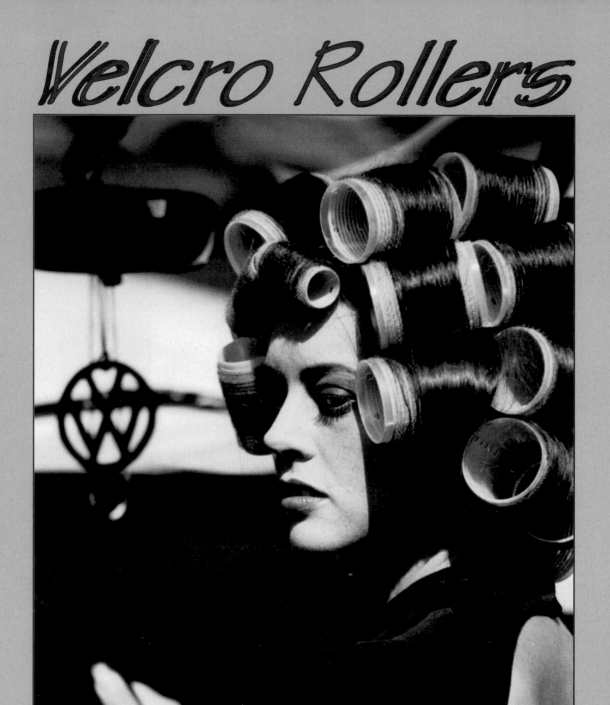

Velcro Rollers quickly produce loose curls in any desired size.

1   Take a 2"-wide, 1"-deep section of hair. Spray with a light hair spray from root to ends.

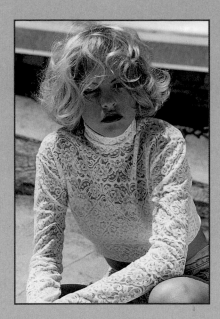

2   Bring section of hair straight out from scalp.

3   Smooth section of hair with roller from roots to ends. Place roller at ends of hair. Using medium tension on hair, roll down to scalp.

4   Repeat process for all desired hair. Allow hair to dry for 10 to 20 minutes or use a blow dryer for five minutes.

5   Slide rollers out of hair and style as desired.

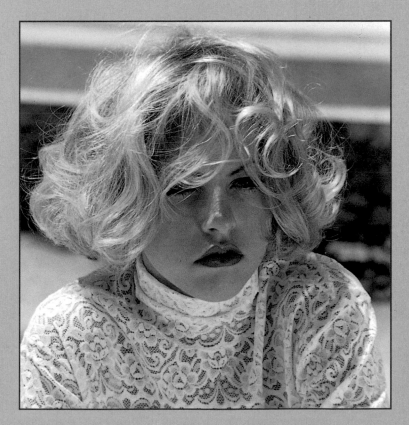

Curling Ropes

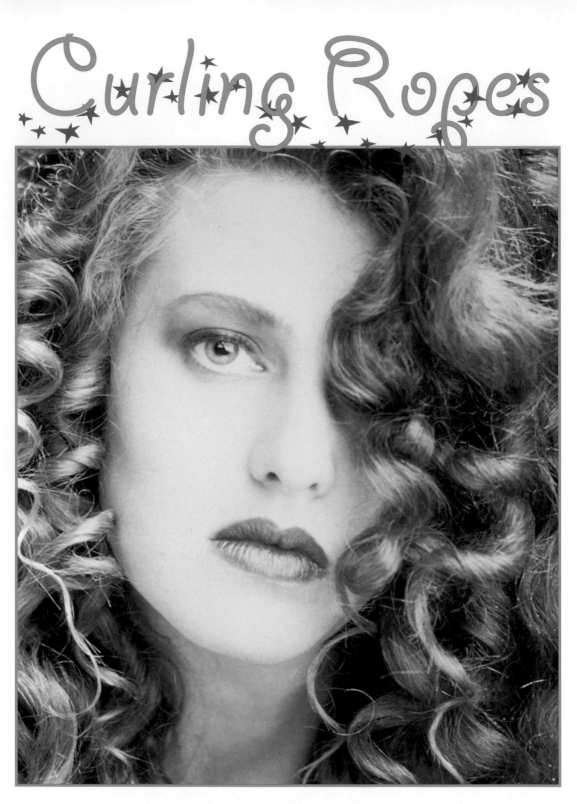

Curling Ropes produce a style with maximum volume and a lot of curls. To make Curling Ropes follow instructions on page 11.

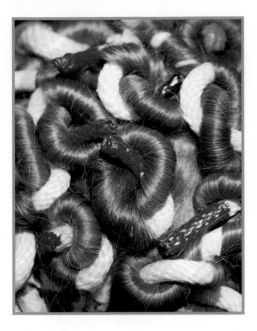

1 Take large square sections or rectangular sections, 1" to 1½" wide, of hair. Apply a light hair spray to hair from roots to ends.

2 Wrap ends of hair with tissue paper or end papers. Start wrapping hair around rope from top end spiralling down. Allow hair to be exposed all the way down rope.

3 Tie rope in a knot to hold. Allow hair to dry under a dryer for 10 minutes or use a blow dryer for 15 to 20 minutes.

4 Undo knot and spin rope out of hair.

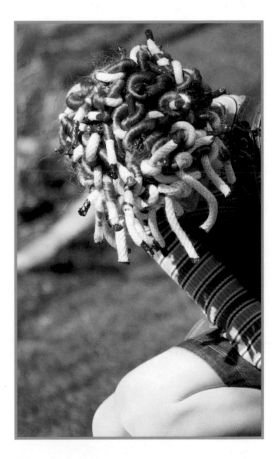

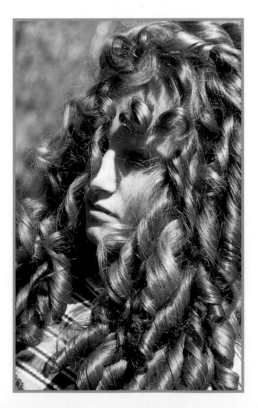

5 Curls should look similar to those in left photo before being styled. Use pick or fingers to style hair.

pONytAil

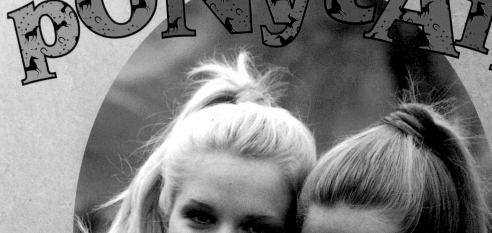

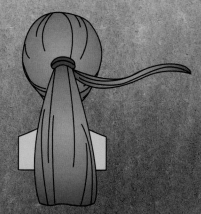

1

Gather hair into a ponytail at desired location on head. Secure with an elastic band. Slip a finger through one section of elastic band. Pull strand of hair out from underside of ponytail.

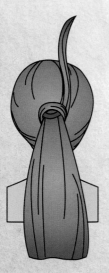

2

Wrap strand around ponytail two or three times depending on hair length. Pull strand of hair down and through elastic band.

3

Move strand of hair around under elastic band until it hangs under ponytail.

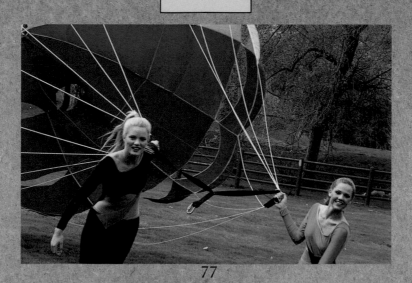

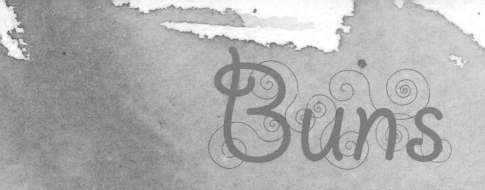

Buns

Helpful Hints

• Start with ponytail high on head for a high bun.

• Start with ponytail on back of head for a back bun.

• Allow hair to fall toward head before twisting for a loose bun.

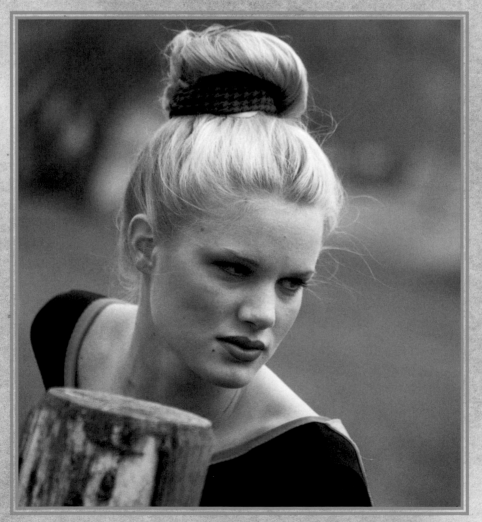

This style is a high bun.

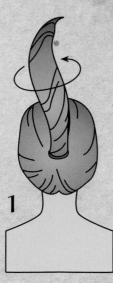

1 Gather hair in a ponytail at desired location on head. Secure with an elastic band. Twist entire ponytail.

This style is a loose bun.

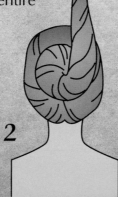

2 Tightly coil ponytail around itself.

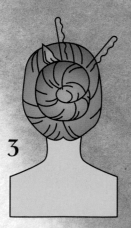

3 Secure bun with hairpins.

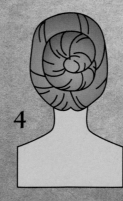

4 Tuck ends under and secure with hairpins.

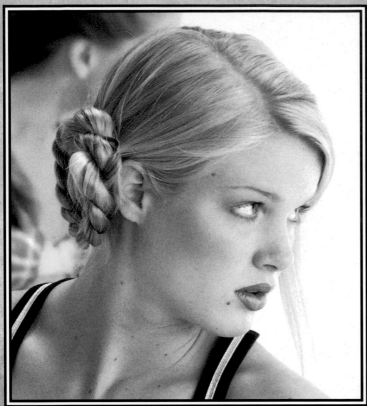

This style is created by coiling two Rope Braids (page 54) into low buns on each side of the head. Only one braided bun is visible in the photo.

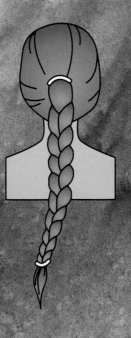

1

Gather hair and place in a ponytail at desired location on head. Secure with an elastic band. Braid ponytail with the Basic Braid (page 24). Secure braid with an elastic band.

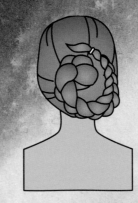

2

Coil braid around itself into a bun. Use bobby pins to secure ends.

This style is created by creating two Braided Buns. Hair is placed in two ponytails—one on each side of the head above the ear, and then braided. Ends are pulled out through the middle of buns instead of tucked into them.

This style is created by making two French Braids (page 28)—one on each side of the back of the head. Each is braided three to five rounds and finished with the Basic Braid (page 24). Each braid is made into a bun. Ends are pulled out through the lower part of buns. If diagonal parts are desired, make them before braiding.

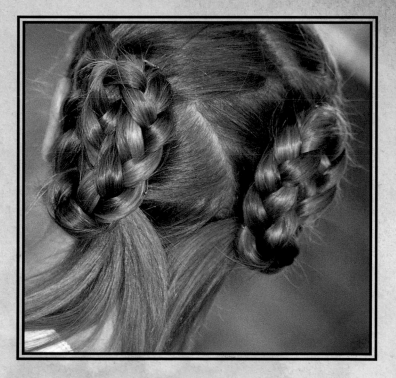

KNOTS

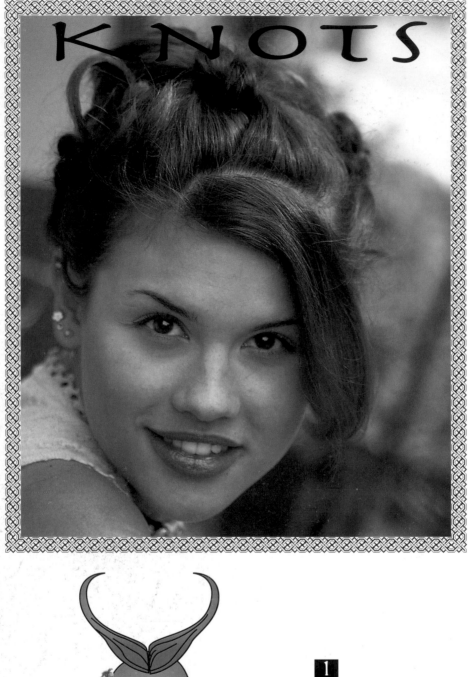

1

Part hair into 1" sections.
Divide section of hair in half.

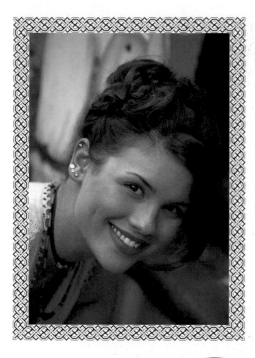

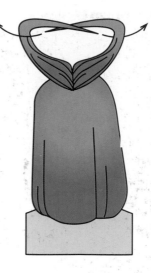

2
Cross ends of hair. Slip one end through opening. Pull gently on each end.

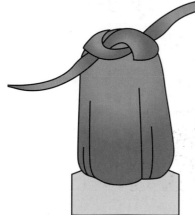

3
Repeat step 2 on the same section of hair.

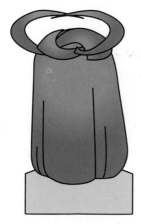

4
Repeat steps 1–3 until all hair is knotted. Place bobby pins in the middle of knots to secure.

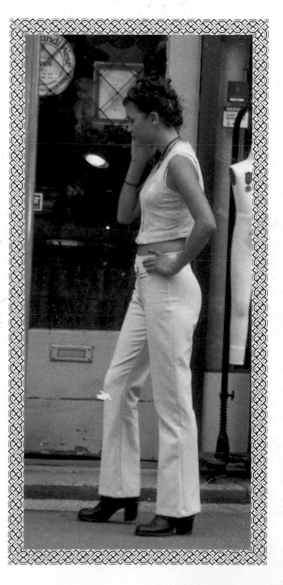

Half Tuck

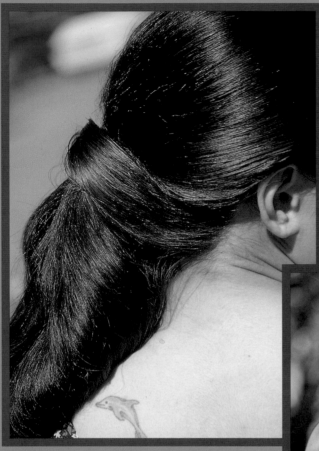

One variation of this style is the Flip Through. Pull ponytail all the way through opening. Another variation of this style is the Full Tuck. Follow steps 1-5 but do not pull any of ponytail through. Use a barrette to pull hair together above the tuck.

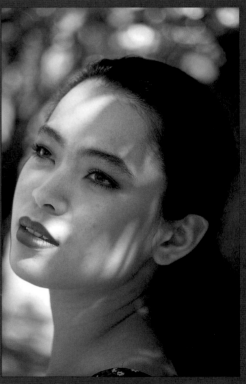

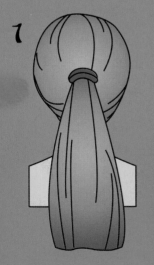

1 Gather hair into ponytail on back of head. Secure with an elastic band.

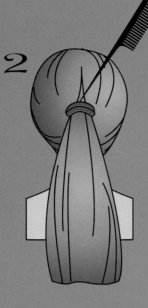

2 Use a long-tailed comb to split ponytail in middle above elastic band.

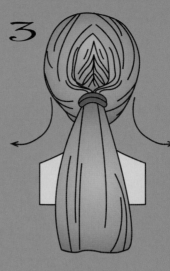

3 Use fingers to make a small opening above ponytail.

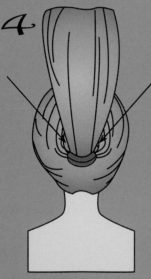

4 Lift ponytail upward.

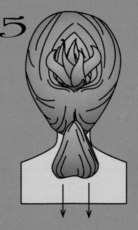

5 Tuck entire ponytail down into opening. Pull half of ponytail through opening.

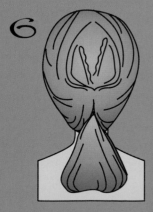

6 Push elastic band and ends down into opening if they are showing. Use bobby pins above elastic band and underneath hanging tuck to secure.

Roll Roll Roll

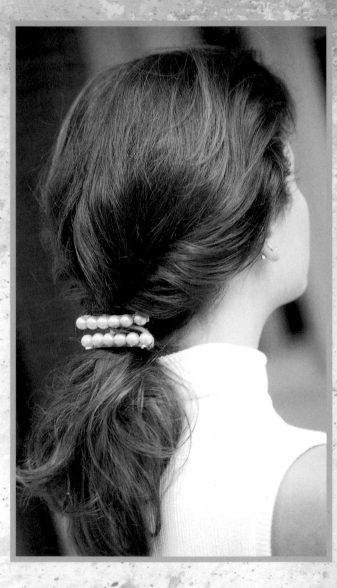

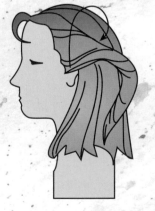

1

Divide hair in half down the back. Clip right section of hair or place over shoulder to keep it out of the way.

2

Take a 1" section above left ear and twist toward back of the head. Hold twist with other hand.

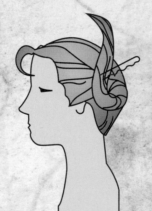

3

Add another section of hair and twist. Gather and twist hair until all hair is added on left side.

4

Give section a few more twists. Clip left side up with other hand.

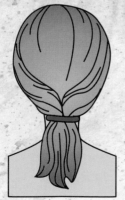

5

Repeat steps 2–4 on right section of hair. Gather sections of hair into ponytail at nape of neck. Secure with a barrette or an elastic band.

A variation of this style is the Braided Roll. Divide hair into three sections. Follow steps 2 and 3, but leave center section untouched. Begin braiding twists by crossing left twist over center section of hair. Then cross right twist over center section forming the Basic Braid (page 24). Secure with an elastic band.

French Twist

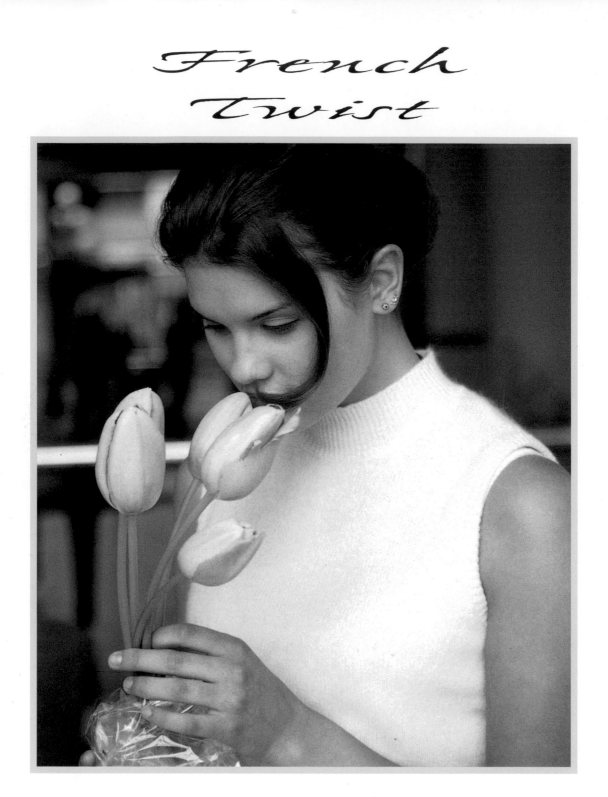

The French Twist works for most hair lengths. It is more difficult to do on very long hair because it is hard to conceal the extra long ends.

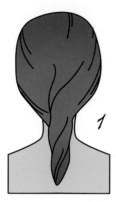

Comb all hair back off the face. (For a softer look, allow a few pieces of hair to fall on face.) Gather hair in a ponytail at nape of neck.

1

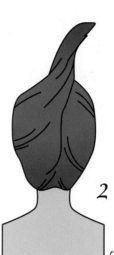

Twist hair counter-clockwise and pull upward with other hand.

2

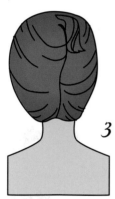

3

Tuck ends of hair inside twist.

4

Secure twist with hairpins.

5   Secure top of twist with a hairpin.

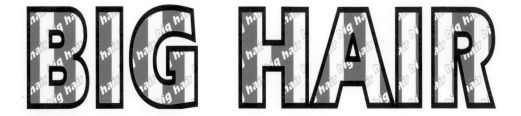

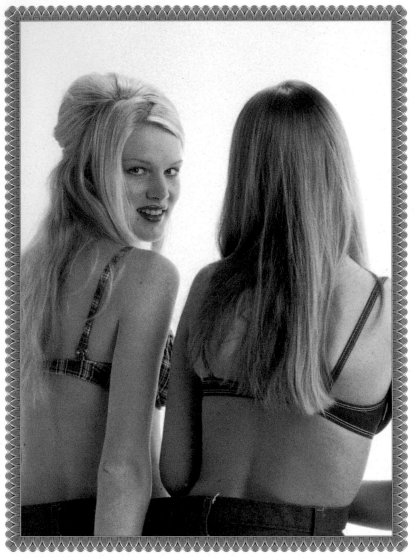

This style is created with hair spray, a long-tailed comb, and a barrette.

1

Section off a 2" parting of hair on crown of head.

2

Tease hair until quite ratted. Lightly spray this section of hair with light hair spray.

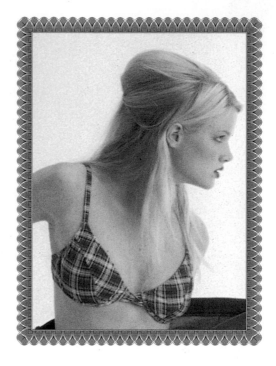

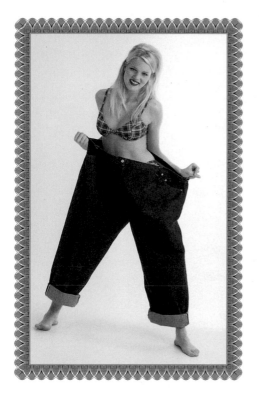

3

Comb a section of hair that is in front of teased hair over top of ratted hair. Spray hair with light hair spray. Part bangs on an angle leaving long side of bangs flat against head.

Parts:

For a dramatic look, choose a zigzag part or a straight-center part. It does not matter where the part is made as long as it is clear and well defined.

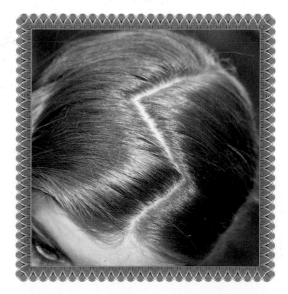

Gelled Twist

This style is created by winding strips of fabric into hair after it has been twisted. Do not saturate hair with gel for this look.

This style is created by twisting two of the three sections up and twisting the last section down. It is secured with barrettes.

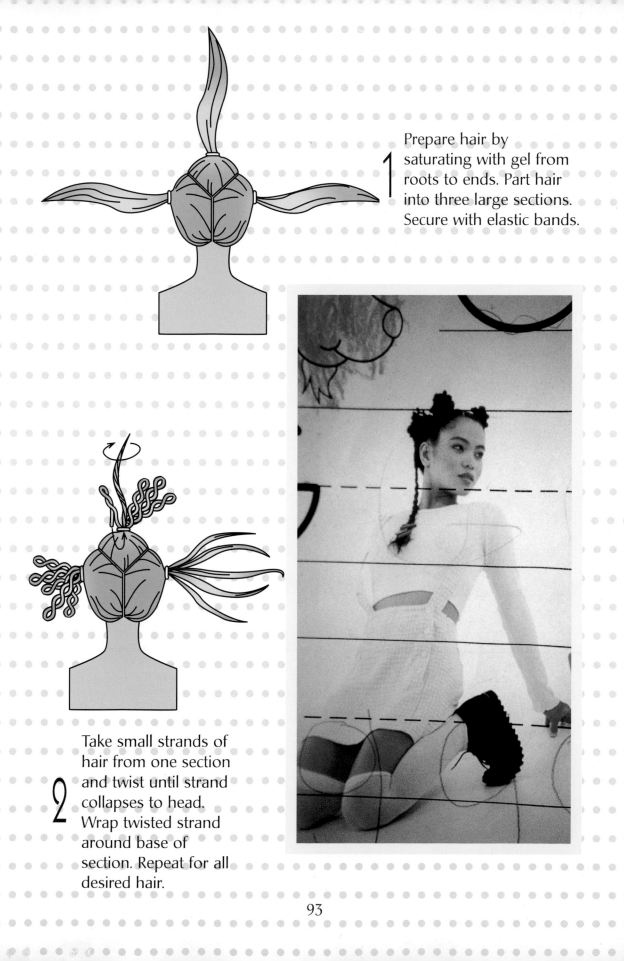

1 Prepare hair by saturating with gel from roots to ends. Part hair into three large sections. Secure with elastic bands.

2 Take small strands of hair from one section and twist until strand collapses to head. Wrap twisted strand around base of section. Repeat for all desired hair.

SCRUNCH & TWIST

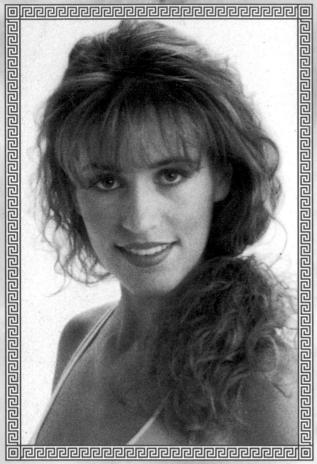

1

Add gel to damp hair from roots to ends Dry hair by scrunching under a diffuser.

2

Take a wide section from behind right ear and slightly twist toward back of head to give height on top. Secure with hair clip.

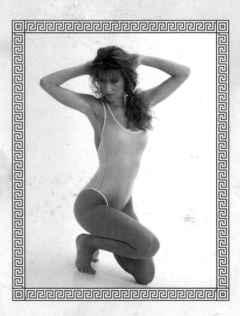

3

Take a wide section from behind left ear and slightly twist toward back of head to give height on top.

4

Remove clip from right side and combine left and right sections of hair. Secure with a barrette or butterfly clip.

CREDITS

Hair: Sherrie Smith, Thomas Hardy, Debbie Hardy, Loretta Brooks, and Pollyanne Barker

Photography: Thomas Hardy

Makeup: Holly Browning

Models: Anita, Pollyanne Barker, Kymberley Benedict, Megan Bouwhuis, ShirleyAnn Cussimanio, Monique Dumas, Shawney Dunn, Lee Figuracion, Amber Grow, Robyn Hardy, Raquel Hurst, Star Jaramillo, Addie King, Danielle Nicholls, and Rachael

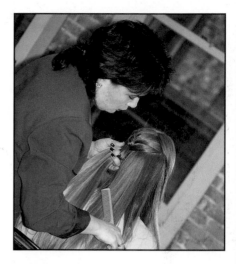

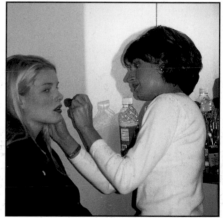

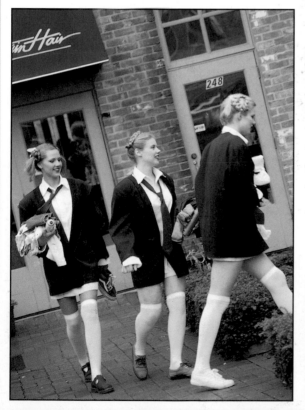

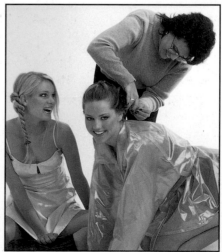

Index

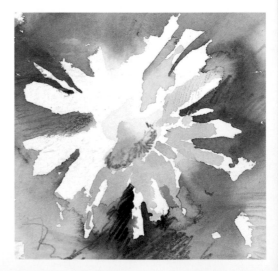